HASHIMOTO'S DIET COOKBOOK

The Ultimate Recipe Book That Contains Easy Delicious Meals For Thyroid Healing

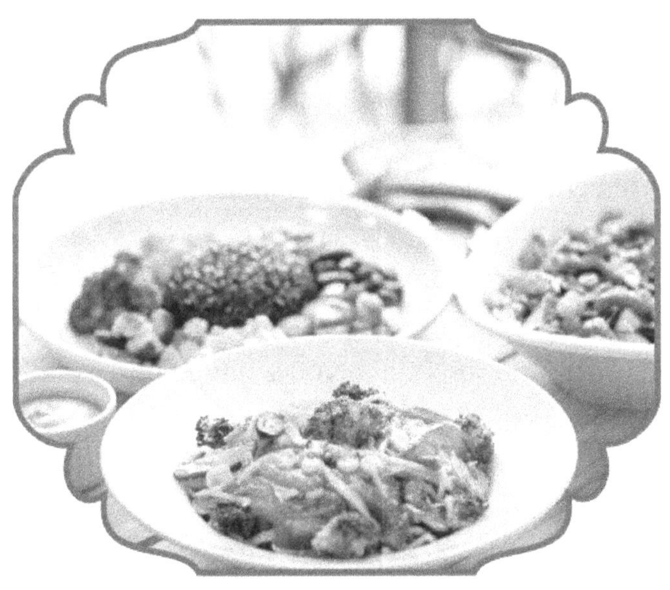

KEVIN S. MAXWELL

Copyright © 2024 by Kevin S. Maxwell

EMAIL ME!

I know that exploring topics that involve food and nutrition can often lead to questions and uncertainty. I invite you to contact me with any questions you may have. I'm here to assist. Please contact me through email at kevinmaxwelldiet@gmail.com and I will try my best to respond to you within 24 hours.

Additionally, if you are interested in exploring other collections of my books. You can check out additional collections of my books by scanning the QR Code that is provided below.

TABLE OF CONTENT

INTRODUCTION

In the quaint town of Serenity Springs, Emma discovered a secret to reclaiming her vitality: a Hashimoto's Diet cookbook that promised to be her ally in healing her thyroid. Plagued by fatigue and unexplained weight gain, Emma's journey toward wellness began as she delved into the pages of this culinary guide.

The cookbook, a treasure trove of nourishing recipes tailored for those with Hashimoto's, unfolded a world where each ingredient was carefully selected to support thyroid health. Emma embraced the vibrant colors and flavors of nutrient-dense meals, realizing that the path to healing lay not in deprivation but in mindful choices.

As she cultivated a newfound culinary prowess, Emma felt the fog of fatigue lifting. The recipes, crafted with an understanding of Hashimoto's complexities, became her beacon of hope. Whole foods, rich in selenium, iodine, and anti-inflammatory properties, adorned her plate, and with each bite, she sensed her body responding with gratitude.

Her energy returned like a long-lost friend, and the stubborn weight began to melt away. Emma revealed in the harmony she felt between her fork and her health, as the cookbook transformed her kitchen into a haven of healing. In the heart of Serenity Springs, Emma's vitality became a testament to the transformative power of a Hashimoto's Diet cookbook — a guide that not only nourished her body but also rekindled the joy of living.

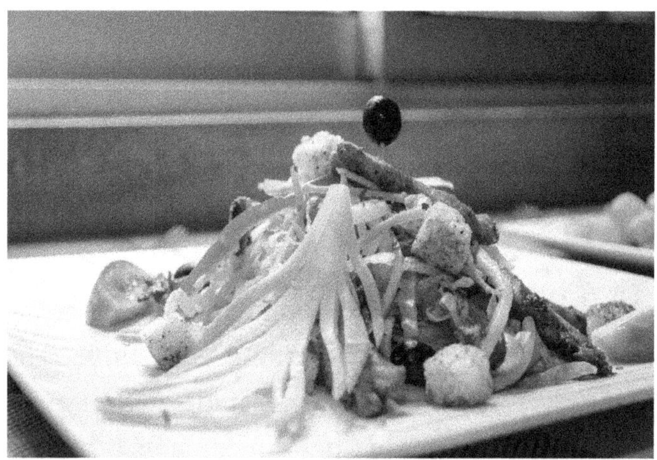

CHAPTER 1: UNDERSTANDING HASHIMOTO'S DIET

The Hashimoto's Diet is a tailored approach to eating designed to support individuals with Hashimoto's thyroiditis, an autoimmune condition affecting the thyroid gland. This specific diet aims to reduce inflammation, support thyroid function, and alleviate symptoms associated with Hashimoto's disease, such as fatigue, weight gain, and mood fluctuations. The Hashimoto's Diet Cookbook becomes an invaluable companion on this wellness journey.

At its core, Hashimoto's Diet focuses on nutrient-dense, whole foods that promote thyroid health. The cookbook, as an extension of this dietary philosophy, serves as a comprehensive guide, offering a diverse array of recipes carefully curated to align with the principles of Hashimoto's Diet. These recipes often emphasize foods rich in selenium, iodine, and anti-inflammatory compounds, crucial for supporting the thyroid and mitigating autoimmune responses.

The cookbook provides a roadmap for individuals to navigate their kitchen with purpose, offering not just meals but a transformative culinary experience. It becomes a tool for empowerment, helping individuals take charge of their health through conscious food choices. By incorporating delicious and nourishing recipes into their daily routine, users of Hashimoto's Diet Cookbook can enjoy a varied and satisfying diet while actively contributing to the healing process.

In essence, Hashimoto's Diet Cookbook is a beacon of support, offering a delightful and practical means for those with Hashimoto's to embrace a lifestyle that fosters both well-being and culinary enjoyment.

CHAPTER 2: HOW TO FOLLOW HASHIMOTO'S DIET

Following a Hashimoto diet involves making mindful and strategic food choices to support thyroid health and manage symptoms associated with Hashimoto's thyroiditis. Here's a step-by-step guide:

1. Educate Yourself: Understand the principles of the Hashimoto's diet. This includes focusing on nutrient-dense, whole foods, and avoiding potential triggers for inflammation. Learn about foods rich in selenium, iodine, and anti-inflammatory properties.

2. Consult with a Healthcare Professional: Before making significant dietary changes, consult with a healthcare professional, especially one experienced in autoimmune conditions. They can provide personalized guidance based on your specific health profile.

3. Emphasize NutrientDense Foods:
Include a variety of fruits and vegetables rich in vitamins and minerals.
Choose lean proteins such as poultry, fish, and legumes.
Incorporate whole grains, nuts, and seeds for fiber and essential nutrients.

4. Be Mindful of Iodine Intake: While iodine is essential for thyroid function, excessive intake may exacerbate Hashimoto's. Consume iodine in moderation and be cautious with iodine-rich foods like seaweed and iodized salt.

5. Prioritize Omega3 Fatty Acids: Include sources of omega-3 fatty acids, such as fatty fish (salmon, mackerel), flaxseeds, and walnuts, to help reduce inflammation.

6. Limit or Avoid Trigger Foods:
Consider reducing gluten intake, as some individuals with Hashimoto's find relief from symptoms by doing so.
Monitor dairy consumption and determine if it affects your symptoms.

7. Manage Stress: Incorporate stress reduction techniques like meditation, yoga, or deep breathing exercises. Chronic stress can exacerbate autoimmune conditions.

8. Keep a Food Journal: Track your dietary choices and note how they make you feel. This can help identify potential trigger foods or patterns that impact your symptoms.

9. Stay Hydrated: Drink plenty of water to support overall health and assist in the elimination of toxins.

10. Consider Supplements: Consult with your healthcare provider about potential supplements like selenium, vitamin D, or omega-3 fatty acids, which may be beneficial for thyroid health.

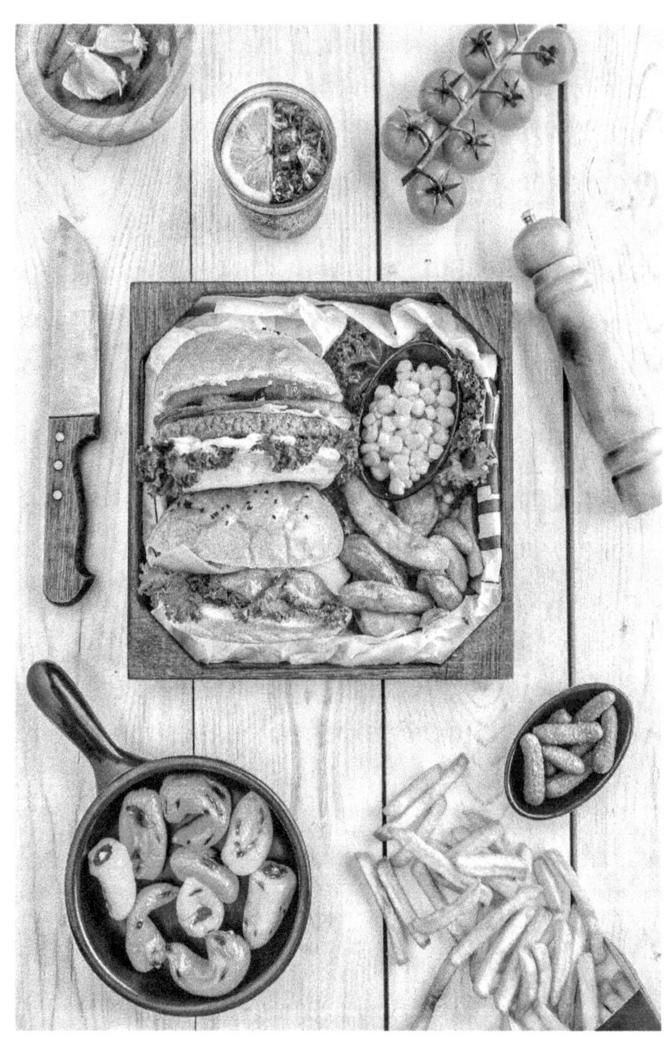

CHAPTER 3: LIST OF INGREDIENTS

Hashimoto's diet focuses on nutrient-dense, anti-inflammatory foods to support thyroid health.

Here are 20 healthy shopping ingredients or lists for a Hashimoto's Diet Cookbook:

1. Leafy Greens:
Spinach, kale, Swiss chard, and collard greens are rich in vitamins and minerals.

2. Cruciferous Vegetables:
Broccoli, cauliflower, Brussels sprouts, and cabbage, are known for their potential anti-inflammatory properties.

3. Lean Proteins:
Chicken, turkey, lean cuts of beef, and fish provide essential amino acids without excessive fat.

4. Fatty Fish:
Salmon, mackerel, and trout are high in omega-3 fatty acids, beneficial for reducing inflammation.

5. Quinoa:
A gluten-free whole grain rich in protein and fiber.

6. Sweet Potatoes:
Packed with vitamins and fiber, sweet potatoes are a nutritious alternative to regular potatoes.

7. Berries:
Blueberries, strawberries, and raspberries are antioxidants that may help combat inflammation.

8. Nuts and Seeds:
Almonds, walnuts, chia seeds, and flax seeds are good sources of healthy fats and essential nutrients.

9. Avocado:
A nutrient-dense fruit with healthy monounsaturated fats.

10. Coconut Oil:
A versatile cooking oil that may have anti-inflammatory properties.

11. Turmeric:
Contains curcumin, known for its anti-inflammatory and antioxidant effects.

12. Ginger:
Has potential antiinflammatory properties and adds flavor to dishes.

13. ProbioticRich Foods:
Greek yogurt, kefir, and fermented foods like sauerkraut support gut health.

14. Bone Broth:
Rich in collagen and nutrients that may promote gut healing.

15. Garlic:
Adds flavor and may have immune-boosting properties.

16. Green Tea:
Contains antioxidants and may support overall health.

17. Mushrooms:
Rich in selenium and may have immune-modulating effects.

18. Organic, PastureRaised Eggs:
A good source of protein and essential nutrients.

19. Hemp Seeds:
Provide omega-3 and omega6 fatty acids along with protein.

20. NonDairy Alternatives:
Almond milk, coconut milk, or hemp milk for those who may be sensitive to dairy.

CHAPTER 4: HEALTHY RECIPES

Turmeric-Ginger Carrot Soup

Ingredients:

- Carrots (1 lb, chopped)
- Onion (1, diced)
- Garlic (2 cloves, minced)
- Turmeric powder (1 tsp)
- Ginger (1 tbsp, grated)
- Vegetable broth (4 cups)
- Coconut milk (1 cup)
- Olive oil (2 tbsp)
- Salt and pepper to taste

Instructions:

1. In a pot, sauté onions and garlic in olive oil until softened.
2. Add chopped carrots, turmeric, and grated ginger. Cook for 5 minutes.
3. Pour in vegetable broth and simmer until carrots are tender.

4. Blend the mixture until smooth, then stir in coconut milk.

5. Season with salt and pepper. Serve hot.

Salmon and Quinoa Bowl

Ingredients:
- Salmon fillets (2)
- Quinoa (1 cup, cooked)
- Broccoli florets (1 cup)
- Cherry tomatoes (1 cup, halved)
- Avocado (1, sliced)
- Lemon (1, juiced)
- Olive oil (2 tbsp)
- Dill (1 tbsp, chopped)
- Salt and pepper to taste

Instructions:
1. Grill or bake salmon until cooked through.

2. In a bowl, combine quinoa, broccoli, cherry tomatoes, and avocado.

3. Drizzle with olive oil, and lemon juice, and sprinkle with dill.

4. Top with cooked salmon. Season with salt and pepper.

Roasted Brussels Sprouts with Walnuts

Ingredients:

- Brussels sprouts (1 lb, halved)
- Walnuts (1/2 cup, chopped)
- Olive oil (3 tbsp)
- Balsamic vinegar (2 tbsp)
- Garlic powder (1 tsp)
- Thyme (1 tsp, dried)
- Salt and pepper to taste

Instructions:

1. Preheat the oven to 400°F (200°C).
2. Toss Brussels sprouts and walnuts with olive oil, balsamic vinegar, garlic powder, thyme, salt, and pepper.
3. Spread on a baking sheet and roast for 20-25 minutes, stirring halfway.

Greek Chicken Salad

Ingredients:

- Chicken breasts (2, grilled and sliced)
- Romaine lettuce (1 head, chopped)
- Cucumber (1, diced)

- Cherry tomatoes (1 cup, halved)
- Red onion (1/2, thinly sliced)
- Kalamata olives (1/2 cup)
- Feta cheese (1/4 cup, crumbled)
- Greek dressing (1/4 cup)
- Lemon (1, juiced)
- Oregano (1 tsp, dried)
- Salt and pepper to taste

Instructions:

1. In a large bowl, combine lettuce, cucumber, cherry tomatoes, red onion, olives, and feta.
2. Top with grilled chicken slices.
3. In a small bowl, whisk together Greek dressing, lemon juice, oregano, salt, and pepper.
4. Drizzle dressing over the salad and toss gently. Serve chilled.

Mushroom and Spinach Quiche

Ingredients:
- Gluten-free pie crust
- Eggs (4)
- Almond milk (1 cup)
- Mushrooms (1 cup, sliced)
- Spinach (1 cup, chopped)
- Onion (1, diced)
- Garlic (2 cloves, minced)
- Nutritional yeast (2 tbsp)
- Olive oil (2 tbsp)
- Salt and pepper to taste

Instructions:
1. Preheat the oven to 375°F (190°C).
2. In a skillet, sauté mushrooms, spinach, onion, and garlic in olive oil until softened.
3. Whisk together eggs and almond milk in a bowl. Stir in nutritional yeast, salt, and pepper.

4. Place the sautéed vegetables in the pie crust, then pour the egg mixture over them.
5. Bake for 35-40 minutes or until the center is set.

Cauliflower Fried Rice

Ingredients:
- Cauliflower rice (4 cups)
- Shrimp or tofu (1 cup, cooked)
- Mixed vegetables (1 cup, diced)
- Scallions (4, chopped)
- Garlic (2 cloves, minced)
- Coconut aminos (2 tbsp)
- Sesame oil (1 tbsp)
- Ginger (1 tsp, grated)
- Eggs (2, scrambled)
- Salt and pepper to taste

Instructions:
1. In a large skillet, sauté garlic, scallions, and ginger in sesame oil.
2. Add mixed vegetables and cook until tender.

3. Stir in cauliflower rice, cooked shrimp or tofu, and scrambled eggs.
4. Drizzle with coconut aminos and season with salt and pepper.

Baked Apples with Cinnamon and Walnuts

Ingredients:
- Apples (4, cored and halved)
- Walnuts (1/2 cup, chopped)
- Cinnamon (1 tsp)
- Maple syrup (2 tbsp)
- Coconut oil (2 tbsp, melted)

Instructions:
1. Preheat the oven to 375°F (190°C).
2. In a bowl, mix chopped walnuts, cinnamon, maple syrup, and melted coconut oil.
3. Fill each apple half with the walnut mixture.
4. Bake for 20-25 minutes or until apples are tender.

Chia Seed Pudding with Berries

Ingredients:

- Chia seeds (1/4 cup)
- Almond milk (1 cup)
- Berries (1/2 cup)
- Vanilla extract (1 tsp)
- Maple syrup (1 tbsp, optional)

Instructions:

1. Mix chia seeds, almond milk, vanilla extract, and maple syrup (if using) in a jar. Stir well.
2. Refrigerate for at least 2 hours or overnight.
3. Before serving, top with fresh berries.

Lemon Garlic Roasted Asparagus

Ingredients:

- Asparagus spears (1 lb)
- Olive oil (2 tbsp)
- Garlic (3 cloves, minced)
- Lemon (1, juiced)

- Salt and pepper to taste

Instructions:
1. Preheat the oven to 400°F (200°C).
2. Toss asparagus with olive oil, minced garlic, lemon juice, salt, and pepper.
3. Roast for 15-20 minutes or until asparagus is tender.

Coconut-Berry Smoothie Bowl

Ingredients:
- Mixed berries (1 cup, frozen)
- Coconut milk (1/2 cup)
- Spinach (1 cup, fresh)
- Chia seeds (1 tbsp)
- Unsweetened shredded coconut (2 tbsp)
- Almond butter (1 tbsp)
- Granola (for topping)

Instructions:
1. Blend frozen berries, coconut milk, spinach, chia seeds, and almond butter until smooth.

2. Pour into a bowl and top with shredded coconut and granola.

Spaghetti Squash with Pesto and Cherry Tomatoes

Ingredients:
- Spaghetti squash (1, halved and seeds removed)
- Cherry tomatoes (1 cup, halved)
- Basil pesto (1/4 cup)
- Pine nuts (2 tbsp, toasted)
- Olive oil (2 tbsp)
- Garlic (1 clove, minced)
- Salt and pepper to taste

Instructions:
1. Preheat the oven to 375°F (190°C).
2. Place spaghetti squash halves on a baking sheet, and cut side up.
3. Drizzle with olive oil and season with salt and pepper.
4. Roast for 40-45 minutes or until squash is fork-tender.

5. Scrape the squash with a fork to create "spaghetti" strands.
6. Toss with cherry tomatoes, pesto, and toasted pine nuts.

Lentil and Vegetable Soup

Ingredients:
- Lentils (1 cup, dried and rinsed)
- Carrots (2, diced)
- Celery (2 stalks, diced)
- Onion (1, diced)
- Garlic (3 cloves, minced)
- Vegetable broth (6 cups)
- Bay leaves (2)
- Thyme (1 tsp, dried)
- Olive oil (2 tbsp)
- Salt and pepper to taste

Instructions:
1. In a large pot, sauté onions, garlic, carrots, and celery in olive oil until softened.
2. Add lentils, vegetable broth, bay leaves, and thyme. Bring to a boil, then simmer until lentils are tender.

3. Season with salt and pepper. Remove bay leaves before serving.

Almond Flour Banana Bread

Ingredients:
- Almond flour (2 cups)
- Ripe bananas (3, mashed)
- Eggs (3)
- Coconut oil (1/4 cup, melted)
- Baking soda (1 tsp)
- Cinnamon (1 tsp)
- Vanilla extract (1 tsp)
- Salt (1/4 tsp)

Instructions:
1. Preheat the oven to 350°F (175°C).
2. In a bowl, mix almond flour, mashed bananas, eggs, melted coconut oil, baking soda, cinnamon, vanilla extract, and salt.
3. Pour the batter into a greased loaf pan.
4. Bake for 45-50 minutes or until a toothpick comes out clean.

Cucumber and Avocado Salad

Ingredients:

- Cucumbers (2, sliced)
- Avocado (1, diced)
- Cherry tomatoes (1 cup, halved)
- Red onion (1/2, thinly sliced)
- Fresh dill (2 tbsp, chopped)
- Olive oil (2 tbsp)
- Lemon (1, juiced)
- Salt and pepper to taste

Instructions:

1. In a bowl, combine sliced cucumbers, diced avocado, cherry tomatoes, red onion, and fresh dill.
2. Drizzle with olive oil and lemon juice. Season with salt and pepper. Toss gently before serving.

Pumpkin and Sage Risotto

Ingredients:

- Arborio rice (1 cup)
- Pumpkin puree (1/2 cup)
- Vegetable broth (4 cups)
- Shallots (2, minced)
- Sage leaves (8-10)
- White wine (1/2 cup)
- Parmesan cheese (1/4 cup, grated)
- Olive oil (2 tbsp)
- Salt and pepper to taste

Instructions:

1. In a pan, sauté minced shallots and sage leaves in olive oil until fragrant.
2. Add Arborio rice and cook until lightly toasted.
3. Pour in white wine and cook until mostly absorbed.
4. Gradually add vegetable broth, stirring until rice is creamy and cooked.

5. Stir in pumpkin puree, Parmesan cheese, salt, and pepper.

Zucchini Noodles with Pesto and Cherry Tomatoes

Ingredients:
- Zucchini (2, spiralized)
- Cherry tomatoes (1 cup, halved)
- Basil pesto (1/4 cup)
- Pine nuts (2 tbsp, toasted)
- Olive oil (2 tbsp)
- Garlic (1 clove, minced)
- Salt and pepper to taste

Instructions:
1. In a skillet, sauté minced garlic in olive oil until fragrant.
2. Add zucchini noodles and cook until just tender.
3. Toss with cherry tomatoes, pesto, and toasted pine nuts.

Chickpea and Vegetable Stir-Fry

Ingredients:

- Chickpeas (1 can, drained and rinsed)
- Broccoli florets (2 cups)
- Bell peppers (assorted colors, 1 cup, sliced)
- Snow peas (1 cup)
- Carrots (2, julienned)
- Tamari or coconut aminos (2 tbsp)
- Sesame oil (1 tbsp)
- Ginger (1 tbsp, grated)
- Garlic (2 cloves, minced)
- Green onions (3, chopped)
- Olive oil (2 tbsp)
- Rice or cauliflower rice (for serving)

Instructions:

1. In a wok or large skillet, heat olive oil and sauté ginger, garlic, and green onions.
2. Add chickpeas, broccoli, bell peppers, snow peas, and carrots. Stir-fry until vegetables are tender-crisp.
3. Pour in tamari or coconut aminos and sesame oil. Toss to coat.

4. Serve over rice or cauliflower rice.

Cabbage and Apple Slaw

Ingredients:

- Green cabbage (1/2 head, shredded)
- Red cabbage (1/2 head, shredded)
- Apples (2, julienned)
- Carrots (2, grated)
- Greek yogurt (1/2 cup)
- Dijon mustard (2 tbsp)
- Apple cider vinegar (2 tbsp)
- Honey (1 tbsp)
- Poppy seeds (1 tbsp)
- Salt and pepper to taste

Instructions:

1. In a large bowl, combine shredded green cabbage, red cabbage, julienned apples, and grated carrots.
2. In a separate bowl, whisk together Greek yogurt, Dijon mustard, apple cider vinegar, honey, poppy seeds, salt, and pepper.
3. Pour the dressing over the cabbage mixture and toss to coat.

Lemon Herb Baked Cod

Ingredients:

- Cod fillets (4)
- Lemon (2, sliced)
- Fresh parsley (2 tbsp, chopped)
- Fresh dill (1 tbsp, chopped)
- Garlic (2 cloves, minced)
- Olive oil (2 tbsp)
- Salt and pepper to taste

Instructions:

1. Preheat the oven to 400°F (200°C).
2. Place cod fillets on a baking sheet. Season with salt, pepper, minced garlic, and chopped herbs.
3. Drizzle with olive oil and lay lemon slices on top of each fillet.
4. Bake for 15-20 minutes or until the fish flakes easily.

Blueberry and Almond Flour Muffins

Ingredients:

- Almond flour (2 cups)
- Eggs (3)
- Blueberries (1 cup, fresh or frozen)
- Maple syrup (1/4 cup)
- Coconut oil (1/4 cup, melted)
- Baking soda (1/2 tsp)
- Vanilla extract (1 tsp)
- Salt (1/4 tsp)

Instructions:

1. Preheat the oven to 350°F (175°C).
2. In a bowl, combine almond flour, eggs, blueberries, maple syrup, melted coconut oil, baking soda, vanilla extract, and salt.
3. Spoon the batter into muffin cups.
4. Bake for 20-25 minutes or until a toothpick comes out clean.

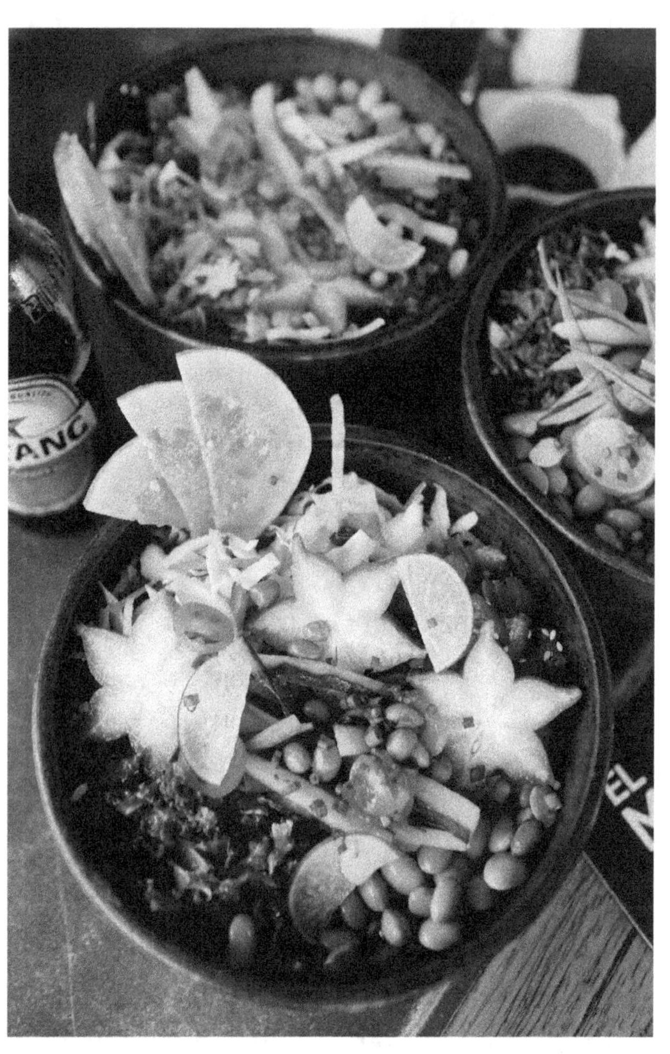

CHAPTER 5: 14-DAY MEAL PLAN

Day 1:
Breakfast: Chia Seed Pudding with Berries
Lunch: Lentil and Vegetable Soup
Dinner: Salmon and Quinoa Bowl

Day 2:
Breakfast: Coconut-Berry Smoothie Bowl
Lunch: Zucchini Noodles with Pesto and Cherry Tomatoes
Dinner: Turmeric-Ginger Carrot Soup

Day 3:
Breakfast: Almond Flour Banana Bread
Lunch: Chickpea and Vegetable Stir-Fry
Dinner: Greek Chicken Salad

Day 4:
Breakfast: Pumpkin and Sage Risotto
Lunch: Cabbage and Apple Slaw
Dinner: Lemon Herb Baked Cod

Day 5:
Breakfast: Blueberry and Almond Flour Muffins
Lunch: Mushroom and Spinach Quiche
Dinner: Roasted Brussels Sprouts with Walnuts

Day 6:
Breakfast: Baked Apples with Cinnamon and Walnuts
Lunch: Cucumber and Avocado Salad
Dinner: Mediterranean Stuffed Acorn Squash

Day 7:
Breakfast: Lemon Garlic Roasted Asparagus
Lunch: Cauliflower Fried Rice
Dinner: Spaghetti Squash with Pesto and Cherry Tomatoes

Day 8:
Breakfast: Chia Seed Pudding with Berries
Lunch: Lentil and Vegetable Soup
Dinner: Salmon and Quinoa Bowl

Day 9:
Breakfast: Coconut-Berry Smoothie Bowl
Lunch: Zucchini Noodles with Pesto and Cherry Tomatoes

Dinner: Turmeric-Ginger Carrot Soup

Day 10:
Breakfast: Almond Flour Banana Bread
Lunch: Chickpea and Vegetable Stir-Fry
Dinner: Greek Chicken Salad

Day 11:
Breakfast: Pumpkin and Sage Risotto
Lunch: Cabbage and Apple Slaw
Dinner: Lemon Herb Baked Cod

Day 12:
Breakfast: Blueberry and Almond Flour Muffins
Lunch: Mushroom and Spinach Quiche
Dinner: Roasted Brussels Sprouts with Walnuts

Day 13:
Breakfast: Baked Apples with Cinnamon and Walnuts
Lunch: Cucumber and Avocado Salad
Dinner: Mediterranean Stuffed Acorn Squash

Day 14:
Breakfast: Lemon Garlic Roasted Asparagus
Lunch: Cauliflower Fried Rice

Dinner: Spaghetti Squash with Pesto and Cherry
Tomatoes

CONCLUSION

In the realm of health and holistic well-being, Hashimoto's Diet Cookbook emerges as a beacon of nourishment, offering a versatile array of recipes meticulously crafted to support those navigating the intricate landscape of Hashimoto's thyroiditis. From the vibrant Greek Chicken Salad to the comforting Turmeric-Ginger Carrot Soup, each dish is a testament to the healing power of mindful nutrition.

This cookbook transcends mere culinary guidance; it becomes a trusted companion on the journey to thyroid health, unlocking a world where flavors marry seamlessly with wellness. The curated selection of ingredients, designed to mitigate inflammation and nurture the thyroid, paints a delicious tapestry of possibilities for every meal.

As you embark on this gastronomic expedition, Hashimoto's Diet Cookbook be your ally. It extends an invitation to savor not just the taste but the transformative potential of each dish. Embrace this culinary adventure as more than a diet – see it as a celebration of your body, a declaration of resilience against autoimmune challenges.

In the embrace of these recipes, find not only vitality but a renewed connection with the joy of living. Let the Hashimoto's Diet be your compass, guiding you towards a path of holistic well-being. Adopt and adapt to this nourishing journey, knowing that every flavorful bite is a step towards revitalizing your body and reclaiming your health.

BONUS: 10 WEEKS MEAL PLANNER/JOURNAL

MEAL PLANNER

Weekly

WEEK

MONTH

MONDAY

SATURDAY

TUESDAY

SUNDAY

WEDNESDAY

SHOPPING LIST

THURSDAY

FRIDAY

MEAL PLANNER

Weekly

WEEK ______________________   MONTH ______________________

MONDAY

SATURDAY

TUESDAY

SUNDAY

WEDNESDAY

SHOPPING LIST

THURSDAY

FRIDAY

MEAL PLANNER

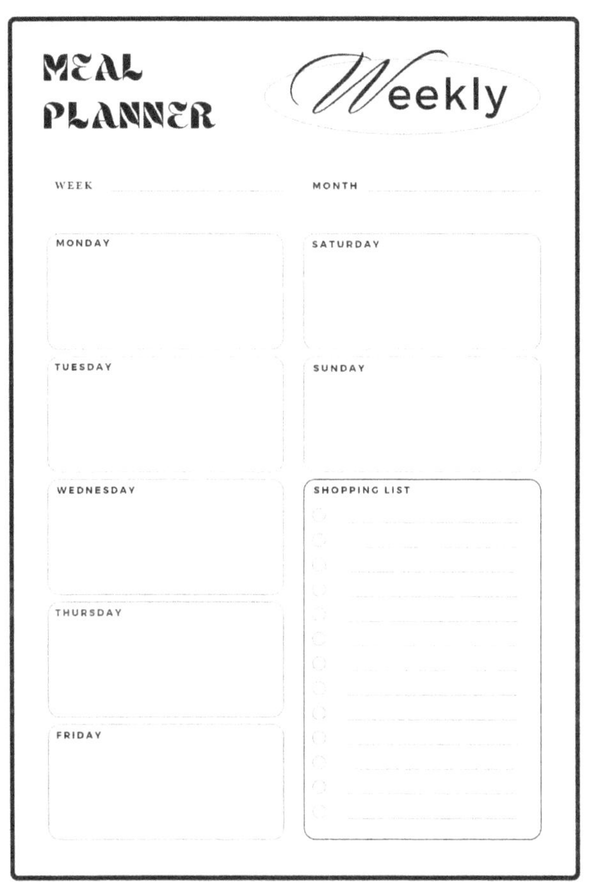

MEAL PLANNER

Weekly

WEEK _________________________   MONTH _________________________

MONDAY

TUESDAY

WEDNESDAY

THURSDAY

FRIDAY

SATURDAY

SUNDAY

SHOPPING LIST

- ○ ______________________
- ○ ______________________
- ○ ______________________
- ○ ______________________
- ○ ______________________
- ○ ______________________
- ○ ______________________
- ○ ______________________
- ○ ______________________
- ○ ______________________
- ○ ______________________
- ○ ______________________
- ○ ______________________
- ○ ______________________

MEAL PLANNER

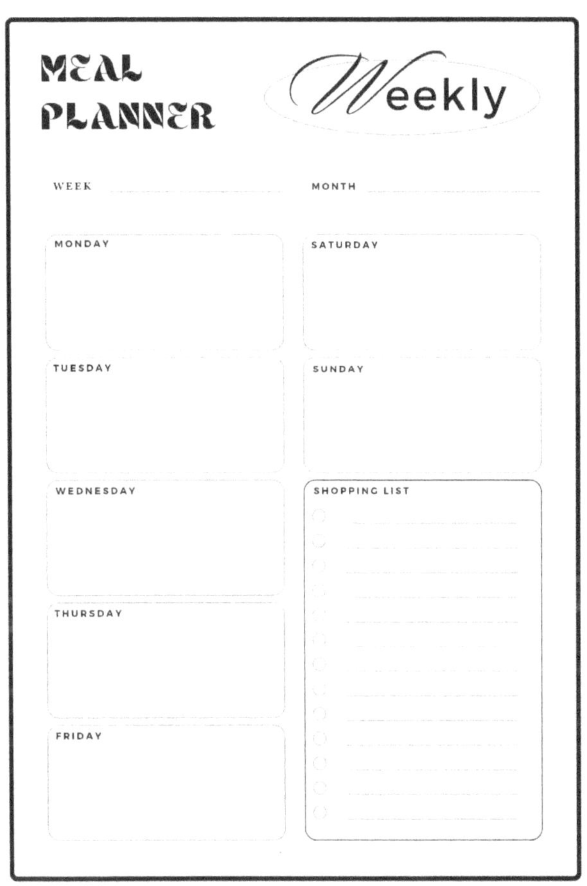

MEAL PLANNER

Weekly

WEEK _______________

MONTH _______________

MONDAY

TUESDAY

WEDNESDAY

THURSDAY

FRIDAY

SATURDAY

SUNDAY

SHOPPING LIST

MEAL PLANNER

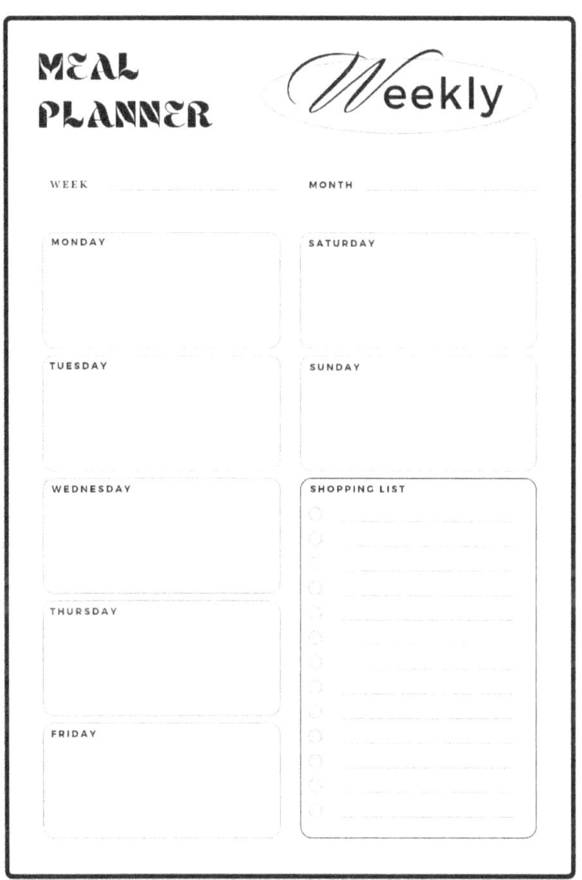

MEAL PLANNER

Weekly

WEEK _______________________

MONTH _______________________

MONDAY

TUESDAY

WEDNESDAY

THURSDAY

FRIDAY

SATURDAY

SUNDAY

SHOPPING LIST

MEAL PLANNER

Weekly

WEEK ....

MONTH ....

MONDAY

TUESDAY

WEDNESDAY

THURSDAY

FRIDAY

SATURDAY

SUNDAY

SHOPPING LIST

MEAL PLANNER

Weekly

WEEK __________________   MONTH __________________

MONDAY

SATURDAY

TUESDAY

SUNDAY

WEDNESDAY

THURSDAY

FRIDAY

SHOPPING LIST